Renew Yourself Thro
and Detoxification D

Womens Wellness Publishing, LLC
www.womenswellnesspublishing.com
www.facebook.com/wwpublishing

Mention of specific companies or products in this book does not suggest endorsement by the author or publisher. Internet addresses and telephone numbers for resources provided in this book were accurate at the time it went to press.

Cover design by Rebecca Rose

ISBN 978-1-939013-91-0

Note: The information in this book is meant to complement the advice and guidance of your physician, not replace it. It is very important that women who have medical problems be evaluated by a physician. If you are under the care of a physician, you should discuss any major changes in your regimen with him or her. Because this is a book and not a medical consultation, keep in mind that the information presented here may not apply in your particular case. In view of individual medical requirements, new research, and government regulations, it is the responsibility of the reader to validate health practices and treatments with a physician or health service.

Acknowledgements

I want to give a huge thanks to my amazing editors Kendra Chun and Sandra K. Friend for their incredibly helpful assistance with putting this book together. I also greatly appreciate my fantastic Creative Director, Rebecca Richards, as well as Letitia Truslow, my wonderful Director of Media Relations. I enjoyed working with all of them and found their help indispensable in creating this exceptional book for women.

Table of Contents

Part I:
Understanding
Detoxification

1

Detoxification is Essential for Your Health

As a physician, I have found that the excessive lifestyle of many of the women patients that I work with takes a real toll on their wellness and, often, contributes greatly to their health issues. Many of my patients tell me that they eat too much unhealthy rich, food and drink coffee or alcoholic beverages in excess of what their bodies can actually handle. This is also true for millions of people in our country.

Many of my patients binge on unhealthy foods when they are feeling stressed, upset, frustrated, or even sad. A big chocolate chip cookie or an ice cream cone looks even more inviting when we need comfort or solace for issues in our lives that are difficult to solve or making us feel unhappy.

Many people also reward themselves with excessive eating for working hard and accomplishing their goals. Binging on rich foods can be a way of patting ourselves on the back for a job well done. In addition, the use of cigarettes, drugs, and alcohol is also very common in order to reduce our level of stress and buffer us from the fears and anxieties that would otherwise dampen our moods. Unfortunately, all of this excess can create a great deal of stress on our bodies.

An additional toxic load on our bodies also comes from many of the modern conveniences that make our lives easier. For example, many chemicals that we are routinely exposed to have potential hazards to our health. This includes spraying the lawn with herbicides instead of digging out weeds, eliminating insects with pesticides, and using toxic solvents for cleaning. Similarly, Western medicine treats most health problems by using drugs to suppress symptoms rapidly but may cause potentially toxic side effects.

All of these pleasures and conveniences of modern living generate enormous amounts of toxic residues that we are exposed to on a daily basis through the air we breathe or even take into our bodies through our skin and mucous membranes.

In order to remain in good health, the body must break down and eliminate all of these toxins on a continual basis. In addition, the body must similarly process the by-products of its own metabolism that, if allowed to accumulate in the body, could cause serious illness or even death. This process is called detoxification and it is one of the most essential processes necessary to keep our bodies healthy and disease free.

Detoxification is one of our body's most essential physiological functions. Detoxification refers to the process of neutralizing or transforming substances that norm-ally would be poisonous or harmful, and eliminating them from the body. Without proper detoxification, toxic substances would accumulate within the body and impair our health by interfering with the function of all our vital organ systems.

Poor detoxification also contributes to many common women's health issues. These include PMS, fibroid tumors, endometriosis, irregular menstrual periods, breast disease, headaches, obesity, heart disease and even women's cancers. An essential part of the healing process for many health conditions is restoring healthy detoxification. I have seen this over and over again with my own patients.

To "jump start" the healing process, many of my patients have expressed interest in juice fasting and detoxification diets. I have given my patients helpful guidelines to facilitate this process so that they could carry out these therapeutic dietary programs successfully and avoid any possible pitfalls.

I have been thrilled with the results of my detox-ification programs for so many of my patients and the benefits have been tremendous. Many women have shared with me that their level of energy and vitality has soared and fatigue and tiredness have disappeared. Women are delighted to find that their skin is clearer and their eyes are brighter and shine with health.

Excess weight disappears, bloating vanishes and immunity is stronger with healthy detoxification. Chronic female health conditions clear up much more readily and health in general is greatly improved. I look forward to you enjoying similar benefits!

I wrote this book to share my guidelines for juice fasting and detoxification with you. I have included sixty delicious juice fasting, modified fasting, and detoxification diet recipes that I have developed. These recipes are not only scrumptious but will help accelerate your journey back to healthy detoxification.

In the first part of this book, I discuss the actual process of detoxification within the body, particularly the metabolism of waste products by the liver. I also discuss how detoxification benefits our health and well-being. In the second part of the book, I share with you useful guidelines on detoxification diets, modified fasting and juice fasting as well as information on nutritional supplements that provide essential support to your liver.

If you are interested in learning about many more nutrient programs and therapies for healthy detoxification, I highly recommend that you read my comprehensive book, *Dr. Susan Lark's Complete Guide to Detoxification.*

2

The Toxins that Assault Our Bodies

Good detoxification produces many health benefits including increased physical vitality and stamina; enhanced mental clarity and acuity; greater ability to remain calm under pressure and increased resistance to illness; good social skills and the ability to get along with other people.

Additional health benefits of detoxification include elimination of toxins from the body, protection of the nervous systems, reduction of the risk of heart disease and female related conditions like PMS, fibroid tumors, endometriosis and breast cancer. It also helps maintain sex drive or libido.

The liver is our primary organ of detoxification. It is the main interface between both ingested and internally created toxins and all the cells of our bodies. If the liver can handle the toxic load we put on our bodies, we can perform at our best and remain healthy. If liver function is impaired, however, performance is negatively affected in many different ways.

Poor detoxification function is linked to muddled thinking, brain fog, chronic low-grade fatigue, or reacting with inappropriate behavior (usually anger) to many of life's inconsequential annoyances.

Two kinds of toxins must be processed by the body, particularly the liver, in order to maintain health: those that are generated in the environment and those that are generated within the body.

Environmental Toxins

Beginning early in this century and accelerating in the last four or five decades, there has been an enormous increase in the number and amount of environmental pollutants that we are exposed to on a daily basis. Our ability to process and excrete these toxins is crucial for survival.

Our bodies are being assaulted on a daily basis by chemicals such as contaminants, pesticides, and herbicides from industrial manufacturing that are in the air, water, and food supply. The amount of toxic chemicals we are exposed to in our environment is staggering.

Each year, the average American is exposed to 14 pounds of food preservatives, additives, flavorings, colorings, waxes (used to preserve produce), anti-microbial agents, along with pesticide and herbicide residues. The U.S. production of synthetic pesticides exceeds 1.4 billion pounds per year. The Environmental Protection Agency (EPA) estimates that there are approximately 70,000 various chemicals in foods, drugs, and pesticides that we may be exposed to, any of which the human body must be prepared to deactivate and remove.

In addition, most of us consume highly processed foods that are laden with artificial chemicals and food additives like MSG (monosodium glutamate), a widely used flavor enhancer; aspartame, an artificial sweetener used in many calorie-reduced foods; and trans fatty acids. These trans fatty acids, which are not found in nature, are polyunsaturated vegetable oils that have been chemically altered by hydrogenation, which converts a fat that is liquid at room temperature into one that is solid, like margarine. All of these artificial chemicals must be detoxified and eliminated by the body.

Toxins also accumulate in the body through the ingestion of addictive substances such as alcohol, caffeine, sugar, and nicotine. Manufacturers promote these addictive substances with billions of dollars of advertising, and many of our social customs support their usage. We have every opportunity to indulge in these substances thanks to daily coffee and cigarette breaks at work and the universal availability of these products in every imaginable channel of distribution.

The body must also detoxify prescription and over-the-counter drugs as well as recreational ones. Drugs are commonly broken down by the liver and eliminated through excretory organs like the kidneys. Many Americans routinely take as many as two to three drugs per day in an attempt to quickly fix a health complaint that is often the result of a poor lifestyle choice. Older Americans have been known to be on ten, twenty, or more, different drugs for various ailments. Over time, this puts enormous strain on the liver. No wonder our livers are overworked and stressed!

Self-Generated Toxins

Beside the toxins we take into our bodies from the outside, our bodies also create endogenous toxins (originating from inside the body), which must also be broken down and eliminated. These are chemicals that we produce internally as by-products of metabolism.

When the detoxification process is efficiently working, these toxins are usually neutralized or excreted without unduly stressing the body. However, if allowed to circulate unaltered through the body, these chemical substances can be highly toxic. For example, when you have a protein-rich meal like a steak dinner, the by-product of the chemical breakdown of the protein is ammonia, which is highly toxic if allowed to accumulate in the body. Normally, ammonia is immediately converted by the liver into a harmless substance called urea that can then be excreted from the body through the kidneys. In patients with severe liver disease, however, this ability to convert ammonia is compromised and ammonia can become elevated to dangerously high levels.

When toxic substances are not properly neutralized and excreted from the body, they are stored in the cells, particularly in fatty tissue. Our cells and tissues can store toxins for months, even years, releasing them during times of low food intake, exercise, or stress. When they are finally released into the bloodstream, the toxins can trigger unwanted symptoms as the body reacts to these poisons, including tiredness, dizziness, nausea, and a racing pulse.

Many chronic and even deadly diseases such as coronary heart disease and diseases of the nervous system, liver, pancreas, and other vital organs have been linked to impaired detoxification. Both the health and performance consequences of poor detoxification have been corroborated by many research studies.

3

How The Liver Detoxifies Waste Products

When the liver is working efficiently, it buffers the body internally from the harmful effects of ingested toxins and environmental pollutants as well as the by-products of our own metabolism. Most people are unaware of the vital role the liver plays in maintaining health, equating it only with a food that tastes good when cooked with onions. However, an understanding of how this vital organ functions is crucial for maintaining high performance levels and overall good health.

The liver is one of the most metabolically active and complex organs in the body. It is also the largest organ in your body, normally weighing about four pounds. The liver lies in the upper right portion of the abdominal cavity beneath the diaphragm. Its large size reflects the multiple functions it performs. It carries out hundreds, if not thousands, of enzymatic reactions along numerous metabolic pathways, playing a pivotal role in maintaining health.

The liver is so crucial to health that it is the only organ that can completely regenerate itself when part of it is removed or damaged. Up to 25 percent of the liver can be removed, and it can still perform its tasks. Moreover, its powers of regeneration are awesome: Within a short period of time, the liver will grow back to its original shape and size.

The liver deactivates and removes the toxic chemicals that circulate throughout the body by two methods. The first method consists of filtering channels called sinusoids. Cells that line the sinusoids surround and break down toxic chemicals, bacteria, and foreign debris via phagocytosis, the process in which one molecule digests another. The second method consists of an extensive two-step system of enzymes that facilitate the deactivation and elimination of toxins.

There Are Two Phases to This Process

In this section, I discuss these two phases. This material is more technical, but it's worth reading if you would like to better understand these processes. Phase I involves a group of enzymes called the cytochrome P-450 system. This system contains between fifty and a hundred enzymes, each of which detoxifies specific types of chemicals. In this phase, toxins undergo oxidation and reduction, in which electrons are transferred between molecules. They are also rendered more water-soluble.

Most harmful chemicals, such as alcohol, pesticides, herbicides, and drugs, are fat soluble when they first enter the body, which allows them to be stored in our fatty tissue and therefore makes them more difficult to eliminate from the body. When toxins are rendered water soluble, they can be more easily excreted through the kidneys and intestinal tract. Phase I of the detoxification process reduces the toxicity of chemicals that would be harmful to the body if they were allowed to remain in their original state.

After this phase, toxins are neutralized, excreted from the body through the intestines or urinary tract, or converted into an intermediate form suitable for further processing by the phase II detoxification system. As these intermediate products are formed, free radicals are generated, and antioxidants are necessary to keep these free radicals from damaging the liver.

Because these intermediate products are potentially dangerous, it is important that phase II of detox-ification be functioning properly to be able to complete the metabolism of these toxins. Foods such as broccoli, Brussels sprouts, cabbage, oranges, tangerines, dill, and caraway seeds can support this function. Broccoli, Brussels sprouts, and cabbage contain indole-3-carbinol and oranges, tangerines, dill, and caraway seeds contain limonene, both of which stimulate the phase I detoxification enzymes.

In Phase II of the detoxification process, the intermediate compounds generated in phase I are transformed into harmless metabolites (breakdown products) that can then be excreted by the body. Phase II enzymes act directly on toxic substances through a process called conjugation, in which these substances are bound with a protective compound. This process either inactivates or neutralizes the toxins or enables them to be more readily eliminated from the body.

Phase II detoxification occurs through the production of glutathione, a substance composed of three amino acids, cysteine, glutamic acid, and glycine, and other sulfur-containing compounds such as sulfuric and glucuronic acid. Several amino acids — including glycine, glutamine, arginine, ornithine, and taurine — along with acetyl CoA and methyl groups (which originate from the amino acid methionine), also combine with and neutralize toxins in phase II. Conjugation removes toxins from their free state, in which they could ordinarily cause cellular stress or damage. Conjugated toxins are then excreted through the urinary tract or the intestines.

An example of substances that must be detoxified by the liver are the many hormones produced within the body. Hormones like estrogen, insulin, adrenaline, and testosterone must be efficiently metabolized and excreted from the body. Otherwise, they would accumulate to toxic levels, producing a variety of adverse effects. Hormones circulate throughout the body, being transported in the blood to various tissues and organ systems.

As hormones pass through the liver, they are inactivated by being bound to glucuronic and sulfuric acid and converted to less potent forms. This process of binding hormones with other chemicals makes them unable to attach to the specific hormone receptor sites within the cells. Once hormones have been detoxified by the liver, they are then secreted with the bile into the small intestine and eliminated through the bowels.

The detoxification of alcohol also occurs in the liver. In addition, many medications, insecticides, heavy metals, and nicotine from cigarette smoke are examples of other toxic substances treated by phase II detoxification.

Part II:
Therapeutic Diets and Nutritional Supplements for Detoxification

4

The Detoxification Diet

Because our livers tend to get so overworked and stressed, it is important to follow a dietary program that supports the health and function of your liver and even incorporate periodic fasting. This will help to maintain your ability to detoxify efficiently.

This means eliminating foods that put wear and tear on the liver and stress our bodies such as high fat and sugar laden foods, rich desserts, caffeine, alcohol, fast foods like pizza and cheeseburgers, fried foods, white flour products, and additives. I know this can be tough in the beginning, but it's worth it in terms of the radiant health and energy that you will enjoy. It means eating a diet that is primarily composed of whole, unrefined, high nutrient foods.

These foods should be organic, unsprayed and unprocessed, whenever possible. It is essential to follow a dietary program that emphasizes lighter, easier to digest foods as well as foods that are beneficial for the liver's functioning. I discuss these dietary principles in more detail in this chapter.

I have found that when my patients have followed a diet to support healthy liver function and enhance detoxification, they usually begin to notice a rapid reduction in their physical symptoms of ill health. Their level of energy and vitality usually is increased as well as their mental clarity and sharpness. Feelings of emotional stress, like being on an "emotional roller coaster," start to smooth out. The mood becomes more calm and balanced. The liver responds quickly to a lighter, healthier diet, especially if the intake of toxic substances are is significantly reduced. An added benefit is that you may find that you begin to shed unwanted pounds and that chronic health issues begin to improve.

When you are customizing your own liver detoxification program, it is important to both cleanse the liver and strengthen and restore its functional capacity at the same time. Since powerful reactions such as headaches, fatigue, and even a runny nose can occur with any detoxification program, you must start slowly and gradually work up to suggested levels.

All dietary changes that are made to improve liver function should be done gradually, over several weeks to several months. As with all health programs, you must experiment within known safe ranges to find the levels that work for your individual biochemistry.

I recommend that you eat a vegetarian emphasis diet, with lots of raw foods or lightly steamed foods. Daily meals should incorporate a variety of salads, fresh fruits and vegetables, whole grains, and legumes. These foods, which are made up of simple molecules of starch, cellulose, fruit sugars, antioxidants, and other easy-to-metabolize substances, place minimum stress on the liver.

Some people need a higher intake of protein to maintain their level of energy. If animal protein is desired, small to moderate amounts of easy-to-assimilate fish, free-range poultry and eggs can be added. Oils should be high-quality cold-pressed monounsaturated and polyunsaturated vegetable oils—used only in small amounts in the early stages of recovery. I personally love to use extra virgin olive oil and flaxseed oil.

In terms of your main meal of the day, many people on a detoxification diet do well with their plate divided up between ½ vegetables or salad, ¼ protein and ¼ complex carbohydrates like whole grains. This can vary, of course, based on your own individual dietary needs. Breakfast can includes smoothies, shakes, and nutritious whole grain cereals with ingredients like ground flax meal, which benefit digestion or easily digestible protein based dishes, as needed.

More Specific Information on Diet

Traditional Chinese medicine recommends the use of certain plant-based foods as part of a dietary regimen for restoring liver function. I have found in my clinical practice that the following foods are well tolerated and seem to accelerate the healing of liver-related problems: beets, broccoli, cabbage, Brussels sprouts, turnips, kale, parsley, lettuce, cucumber, green foods such as spirulina, chlorella, and barley grass, beans and peas, sprouts, tofu, rice, millet, and fresh fruits, preferably consumed during the warmer months. However, I recommend avoiding vinegar and citrus fruits if you tend towards over acidity.

In contrast, a diet that includes large amounts of red meat, dairy products, and fatty foods like nuts and chips burden the liver, which must break down the large and more complex structures of these proteins and fats into triglycerides, prostaglandins, and an array of waste products that can be excreted by the body. When the liver cannot process fats, they accumulate inside liver cells, creating fatty degeneration of the liver. In time, these fats will be deposited in the arteries, leading to eventual heart problems and stroke.

As previously mentioned, to decrease stress on the liver, it is also critical to avoid certain substances, such as refined white sugar and flour, alcohol, caffeine, and drugs (other than needed prescribed medicines), because the breakdown of these products leaves toxic residues that the liver must neutralize. Following a lighter, fresher diet allows the liver to go through a gradual self-cleansing process, without causing further stress.

Eat only those foods that do not add to the stress load on the liver. Constantly experiment with the suggested food groups and find those you like and tolerate best. Incorporate these foods into recipes you enjoy or find recipes that use these food groups. Remember, it is virtually impossible to rebuild and restore liver function without eliminating foods that are high in fat and sugar content.

Individuals who are following a program to restore their detoxification capability may still want to enjoy an occasional meal of animal protein. The following suggestions will put the least strain on your liver. Eat eggs prepared simply, either soft- or hard-boiled. Avoid eggs prepared with fats and oils such as deviled or fried eggs. Choose soft-textured, easy-to-digest fish such as salmon, trout and other fish rich in healthful omega 3 fatty acids, which reduce inflammation within the body. It is best to avoid red meat such as pork, lamb, or beef, which are high in saturated fat and more fibrous in texture, and therefore more difficult to digest.

While you are restoring your liver function, eliminate all alcoholic beverages. Switch to mineral water and herbal teas such as chamomile and peppermint, which are therapeutic for the liver. Once liver function is restored, alcohol intake should be limited to an occasional, single beverage.

Individuals with impaired detoxification function should make an effort to avoid eating after 6:00 p.m. or 7:00 p.m. at the very latest. In addition, eat your heaviest meals early in the day, with your last meal being the lightest. This will help to prevent undue stress on the liver during the night when it should be repairing and restoring itself rather than trying to metabolize the residues of a heavy meal. Eating late at night can significantly hinder a liver restoration program. My patients have found that avoiding heavy meals eaten late at night significantly reduces morning grogginess and brain fog.

All dietary changes that are made to improve liver function should be done gradually, over several weeks to several months. Too extreme and rapid a change in one's diet can induce waste products to be eliminated more rapidly than the liver can handle, triggering symptoms like nasal congestion, flulike symptoms, diarrhea, bad breath, and aches and pains.

As with a detoxification diet, you can continue taking any nutritional supplements that you would normally use during a modified fast in order to provide your body with the essential support that it needs.

5

Modified Fasting

Many books on detoxification recommend fasting as the quickest and most efficient way to rid the body of accumulated toxins, but true fasting is very difficult for the average American. A true fast consists of consuming only water or diluted liquids such as juices, broths, or herbal teas for a prescribed period of time.

Fasting has been practiced for thousands of years by people of nearly all cultures throughout the world. Used for purification, penance, during periods of mourning, and to strengthen mental, physical, and spiritual powers, fasting is an ancient practice with modern applications.

However, most of us in the United States live busy, stressful lives, with myriad responsibilities at home, school, and work. We don't often have the luxury of a large block of time without responsibilities to undertake the intensity of a true fast.

Fasting can accelerate the elimination of toxins from the body and trigger a number of uncomfortable symptoms including nasal discharge, headache and flu-like symptoms.

If you are working and active, a true fast can be very disruptive. However, I have found with my own patients that many of them do best with a program of two or three light meals a day.

These meals can consist of fruit and vegetable juices; low-sodium and low-fat broths; fresh shakes and smoothies; herbal teas; light, easy-to-digest solid foods, such as uncooked or lightly steamed organic vegetables and sprouts; and smaller amounts of thoroughly cooked starches, grains, and legumes.

Such a program can be followed for a few days up to several weeks, although some people may choose to do this for an even longer period of time. This program will help to begin to clear toxins from the liver.

You should consume only organic fruits, vegetables, grains and legumes during a modified fast, because if you are trying to eliminate toxins from the body, consuming foods covered with chemical pesticides and fertilizers is counterproductive. Fruit and vegetable juices should be prepared fresh, used within a day or two, and always kept refrigerated.

Some bottled vegetable juices may be used when fresh ones are unavailable. Excellent vegetable juices include carrot, beet and beet green, parsley, celery, cucumber, kale and spinach, but a wide variety of other vegetables can be used for juicing. To enhance the cleansing action of these juices, add a little garlic or wheatgrass juice.

However, don't drink fruit juices by themselves because they are highly acidic and high in concentrated sugars. Fruit juices can be mixed with vegetable juices if you miss the sweet flavor of fruit. If you can't live without some fresh fruit juice, the best ones to use are papaya and melon, preferably diluted by 50 percent with water. But if you are hypoglycemic or suffer from fatigue, you should avoid drinking fruit juice completely. The simple sugars found in fruit juices will cause an overproduction of insulin by the pancreas. This, in turn, will trigger the roller-coaster effect of quick highs and sudden lows in blood sugar levels.

In contrast, eating the whole fruit slows down absorption of the sugar because of the fiber contained within the fruit. In addition, when fruit juices are mixed with protein and oils (like protein powder or ground flaxseed) as is commonly done with smooth-ies, the sugar from the juice is absorbed much more slowly and does not cause a hypoglycemic type of effect.

Smoothies and shakes are great meals to prepare during a detoxification diet or modified fast because they contain the full range of nutrients needed to maintain your level of energy. Yet, they do not put stress on the digestive organs, including the liver, because all of the ingredients are already broken down into small particles and liquefied in a blender, thereby making digestion much easier. I share with you a number of great smoothie recipes in the recipe section of this book that support healthy digestion and detoxification.

You can continue taking any nutritional supplements that you would normally use during a modified fast in order to provide your body with the essential support that it needs.

6

Juice Fasting

If you decide that you want to try a juice fast in which you consume only fruit and vegetable juices while totally abstaining from food consumption, you will have an accelerated cleansing and detoxification of your body. Juice fasting is usually done for one to three days, although some people may choose to fast for a longer period of time. However, if you choose to fast for longer periods of time, you may want to consult with your health care practitioner as to the advisability of doing this, given your particular health status.

Fasting for short periods of time can be beneficial in that it takes stress off of your digestive organs. It is particularly beneficial to the body to stop eating fast food, alcohol, coffee, soft drinks, sugar, refined flour products, fried foods, and all other foods that put excessive wear-and-tear on our systems.

Juice fasting can also help to accelerate weight loss and to release patterns of addiction to sugar, caffeine, soft drinks, and overeating. Some people choose to do juice fasting as part of an alternative health program to support healing from a chronic health issue or as part of a cleansing process to refresh and revitalize their bodies. Juicing can add a wider variety of vegetables and fruits to your diet.

Such rapid detoxification can, however, trigger several troublesome symptoms, including a displeasing taste in the mouth, a thick coating on the tongue, skin odor and/or eruptions, headaches, and digestive upset. A person may develop flu-like symptoms or a nasal discharge for a day or two. Most people who go on a rigorous, traditional fast experience a drop in their energy level and have constant thoughts of food. Some people experience even more serious symptoms, such as faintness or an irregular heartbeat, which should be reported to a physician immediately.

Cautions on Juice Fasting

- If you are a pregnant or nursing woman, you should avoid juice fasting.

- If you are diabetic or suffer from severe hypoglycemia or chronic fatigue, be sure to consult with your physician about the advisability of doing juice fasting.

- If you suffer from anemia, anorexia or low body weight, kidney disease, epilepsy or other pre-existing condition, I recommend that you consult with your own health care provider about the advisability of doing a juice fast.

- If you are using prescription medication, I recommend that you consult with your own health care provider or physician about the advisability of doing a juice fast. Prescription medication should not be discontinued or reduced on your own.

Guidelines for Juice Fasting

- When doing a fast, you should use only freshly juiced organic fruits and vegetable. Do not use commercial bottled or canned juices that are processed, may have been heavily sprayed with pesticides and herbicides and lack the same level of vitality as fresh juices.

- Grapefruit juice should be avoided during a juice fast, especially if you are taking prescription drugs since this can affect the manner in which certain drugs are metabolized in your body.

- You may want to do a modified fast, as outlined in the previous chapter, for several days up to a week before beginning and after completing a juice fast. This will help you prepare for a fast and also assist you in transitioning back to a normal diet.

- Juice should be ingested throughout the day. Many people will choose to drink between 32 to

35   Juice Fasting and Detoxification

64 ounces of juice per day, but amounts can vary from person to person, depending on size and hydration needs. Be sure to also drink spring or filtered water to maintain adequate hydration.

- It is best to do juice fasting during the warmer months and abstain from fasting during the cold winter months when the body needs warmer, more heating foods.

- Before juicing fresh fruits and vegetables, be sure to wash them thoroughly to remove any dirt, pesticides, and herbicides. Some women even wash their fruits and vegetables in a diluted solution of bleach and water if they are concerned about chemical contamination. Leave the skin of the fruit or vegetable intact, when possible, or pare it thinly because many nutrients are concentrated in this part of the plant. And be sure to store fresh vegetables in the refrigerator soon after obtaining them to avoid loss of nutrients.

- You may continue the use of nutritional supplements that you consider to be essential for your health. However, if you are comfortable, you may want to abstain or use an abbreviated number of vitamins and minerals for a few days during the fast.

- While you can continue with your normal routine during the fast, it is best to minimize or avoid doing very strenuous physical or mental activity. A daily walk is beneficial if that it promotes healthy oxygenation and circulation.

- You may also find it beneficial to do cleansing techniques, including colon cleansing, enemas, and dry brush massage. This will help in the elimination of toxins from the body. I discuss these along with many other detoxification therapies in my comprehensive book, *Dr. Susan Lark's Complete Guide to Detoxification*.

Types of Juicers

There are two types of equipment that you can use to make your fresh fruits and vegetable juices: juicers and high speed blenders. I make fresh juice often and have worked with both types of equipment. I have found that they both make excellent quality juices, although the process and the composition of the juicer can vary.

Whatever type of juicer you decide to buy, it is very important to take good care of your equipment. It should be washed and cleaned carefully after use and stored in a dark, cool area.

Blenders

Juicing fruits and vegetables in a blender liquefies the food, breaking all of its components into extremely small particles, and enhances (or replaces) the mechanical digestive step of chewing. The surface area of the food is dramatically increased, thereby eliminating one of the functions of pancreatic and other enzymes in the breakdown process and hence requiring less enzyme production.

Blenderized juice is absorbed and assimilated very easily, with minimal symptoms of incomplete or poor digestion such as bloating, gas, and food remaining in the digestive tract for long periods of time. The nutrients from the food are much more readily available when food is taken in blenderized form.

The entire fruit and vegetable, including the skin and seeds, can be liquefied in a blender thus greatly increasing the range of nutrients present in the juiced form. There is no leftover pulp with its valuable fiber that gets discarded, as with juicers. Because the whole fruit and vegetable is processed, blenderized juices can be more filling than those made by a juicer. These liquid meals can be tremendously beneficial for conditions related to over acidity or low enzyme production such as fatigue, brain fog, inflammatory conditions, autoimmune problems, and even cancer.

You can use any commercially available blender or food processor, however, I have found that Vitamix (vitamix.com) super powerful blenders that can pulverize virtually any whole food into a liquid (in contrast, juicers tend to extract the juice while discarding the nutrient-rich pulp).

Juicers

There are three main types of electric juicers: masticating, centrifugal, and triturating juicers. These juicers vary by the methods that they use to extract the juice from fruits and vegetables.

Masticating –This type of juicer utilizes a single gear driven by a motor. Using this type of juicer is a slower process as it kneads and grinds fruits and vegetables that are placed in a chute. It chews up the plant fiber and breaks down the produce in a spiral rotating process. The masticating juicer is considered to be a higher quality juicer. It produces a greater quantity of juice of excellent quality.

Centrifugal – This type of juicer utilizes a spinning blade that grinds fruits and vegetables and pushes the extracted juice through a strainer. The pulp is separated from the juice so that it can be easily discarded. The juicing process occurs more rapidly than with the masticating juicer. Less juice, however, is usually extracted with a centrifugal juicer so more juice is wasted since it is retained in the pulp.

Triturating – This type of juicer utilizes twin gears and turns at a slower rpm to extract the maximum amount of juice. The process occurs in two steps. In the first step, the fruit and vegetables are crushed, while in the second step the juice is extracted. This process is thought of create a high quality juice, despite the slowness of the process.

Nutrients Found In Fresh Fruits and Vegetables

Fresh fruits and vegetables contain a wide variety of essential nutrients that will be present in their juices that can be of great benefit when doing a fast. In this section, I share with you some of these incredible nutrients to help you choose which fruits and vegetables you may want to include in your juice fast.

Benefits of Fruits

Fruits are an excellent source of vitamin C, which provides important protection against cancer and heart disease. In fact, vitamin C helps protect the cardiovascular system by preventing oxidation of the low-density lipoprotein cholesterol (LDL cholesterol). This is an early event leading to the development of atherosclerosis. Certain cancers, such as cervical cancer, occur more frequently in vitamin C deficient individuals. Vitamin C reduces capillary fragility and can help control or reduce heavy menstrual flow in susceptible women, particularly in teenage girls and in women who are transitioning into menopause.

Vitamin C also has important anti-stress and immune stimulant properties. It is needed by the adrenals for the production of adrenal cortical hormones. Women who are deficient in vitamin C due to low dietary intake or insufficient supplementation tend to handle stress less effectively, resulting in anxiety, nervous tension, and even chronic fatigue.

Adequate vitamin C intake helps us to fight off a wide range of viral and bacterial infections. Vitamin C is also needed for collagen production, which maintains the structural integrity of the skin. The best fruit sources of vitamin C include citrus fruits like oranges, grapefruits, tangerines, and lemons, and other fruits such as melons, strawberries, and other berries.

Citrus fruits and berries are also rich in bioflavon-oids, another essential nutrient that affects blood vessel strength and permeability. Bioflavonoids also have an anti-inflammatory effect, important to women with allergies, menstrual cramps, or arthritis. Many bioflavonoids are natural sources of plant estrogens. Like our own endogenous estrogen, these weak dietary sources of estrogen can be supportive of the female reproductive tract and can improve mood and increase energy levels in women with PMS or menopausal symptoms.

Bioflavonoids can also help relieve estrogen-related migraine headaches. Although citrus fruits are excellent sources of bioflavonoids and vitamin C, they are highly acidic and may be difficult to digest for some women with food allergies or sensitive digestive tracts.

Citrus fruits are used for the commercial production of bioflavonoid supplements. Unfortunately, much of the bioflavonoids in citrus fruits are found in the inner peel and pulp of the fruit. This is the bitter part of the fruit that many people discard, unaware of its health benefits. Also, the skin of grapes, cherries, and many berries are rich sources of bioflavonoids. Make sure to eat the whole fruit rather than just the juice.

Yellow and orange fruits such as cantaloupe, papaya, persimmons, apricots, and tangerines should be included in your diet because of their high vitamin A content. Vitamin A in fruits is available in high levels as a provitamin called beta-carotene. Like vitamin C, vitamin A helps to protect the body from developing many types of cancer, including cervical, lung, and bladder cancer. It also helps to protect the cardio-vascular system from heart attacks and lowers the risk of strokes.

Vitamin A in the form of beta-carotene helps to improve female health in a number of other ways. Deficiencies in vitamin A have been linked to benign breast disease, heavy menstrual bleeding, and skin aging. Because it is needed for healthy mucous membranes, a lack of vitamin A can worsen the signs of aging of the vagina and genitourinary tract after menopause. Vitamin A is also essential for healthy immune function, resistance to infection, and healthy vision. Clearly, beta carotene-containing fruit should be eaten often for adequate intake of this essential nutrient.

All fruits are excellent sources of potassium, though grapefruits, figs, berries, bananas, peaches, apricots, raisins, and melons are particularly rich in this important mineral. Adequate potassium intake is necessary for good health. It helps to regulate fluid balance in the body. When women are deficient in potassium at the expense of high levels of sodium (which is ubiquitous in the American diet as table salt), health problems can occur. Low potassium and high sodium levels can predispose a person to bloating and fluid retention during the premenstrual period.

In women entering menopause, potassium deficiency can worsen fluid retention, weight gain, and high blood pressure. Women with a low potassium intake tend to tire easily and lack stamina and endurance. In fact, several studies have shown when a combination of potassium and magnesium supplements is taken energy levels improve significantly.

Benefits of bananas, to name a few — are good sources of calcium and magnesium. You can eat these fruits often, as their minerals are essential for proper nervous system and muscular function.

In recent years, a special group of exotic fruits have been available through health food stores or through the Internet. These fruits are so rich in their antioxidant content that I call them super antioxidant fruits. These include acai berries, goji berries, noni, and mangosteen.

In case you don't know what an antioxidant is, let me explain. An antioxidant is a substance that protects our bodies from free radical damage. A free radical is a type of oxygen molecule that freely moves inside cells, reacting with proteins, fats, and DNA, changing and damaging their structure and disrupting their functions. Free radicals are generated by the metabolism of oxygen and other chemicals, including cigarette smoke, unsaturated fats, food additives, and environmental chemicals — and even by aerobic exercise. Free radicals can cause an extreme amount of damage within our bodies.

Antioxidants help to protect us from free radical damage. Antioxidants unite with free radicals and deactivate them, preventing them from doing damage. A variety of substances have an antioxidant function, including beta carotene, vitamin C, vitamin

A, vitamin E, selenium, and glutathione. It is important to either include all of the antioxidants in the diet or take them as supplements.

Super antioxidant fruits contain a high content of anthocyanins, which are a subcategory of plant bioflavonoids. These are the pigments that give these fruits their strong, beautiful colors like reds and purples and are also protective antioxidants.

Super fruits like pomegranate are also a rich source of other antioxidants like polyphenols, some of which have anti-inflammatory benefits. Early research on pomegranate juice suggests that it may improve blood flow to the heart is people with coronary heart disease. It may also be beneficial in slowing the growth of prostate cancer, according to research from UCLA. There are benefits for women, too, in eating pomegranates. It contains plant estrogens that have been found to be useful in relieving vaginal dryness.

Types of Fruits

Temperate Climate Fruits
Apples
Pears
Peaches
Nectarines
Apricots
Plums

Citrus Fruits
Grapefruit
Lemons
Limes
Oranges
Tangelos
Tangerines

Cherries
Bing
Queen Anne

Melons
Cantaloupe
Casabas
Persian honeydews
Watermelons

Grapes
Red seedless
Thompson seedless

Berries
Blackberries
Blueberries
Boysenberries
Cranberries
Gooseberries
Lingonberries
Raspberries
Strawberries

Tropical and Subtropical Fruits
Avocados
Bananas
Coconut
Guavas
Kiwis
Papayas
Pineapples

Super Antioxidant Fruits
Acai berry
Goji berry
Mangosteen
Noni Berry
Pomegranate

Benefits of Vegetables

In the past few decades, many research studies have concluded that the nutrients found in vegetables play an important role in protecting us from health problems. These essential nutrients include vitamin A, vitamin C, calcium, magnesium, potassium, iron, iodine, and more. In addition, vegetables contain other chemicals that help protect against heart attacks and boost immune function. Starchy vegetables help regulate blood sugar levels.

The form of vitamin A found in foods is beta-carotene, a provitamin, which is converted to vitamin A once it's taken into the body through the diet by the liver and intestines. Beta carotene is found in high doses in fruits and vegetables and is quite safe. For example, one glass of carrot juice or a sweet potato, each contain 20,000 IU of beta-carotene. Many people eat two to three times this amount in their daily diet. In contrast, high doses of supplemental vitamin A derived from fish liver oil can accumulate in the liver to toxic levels.

Vegetables high in vitamin A tend to have an orange, red, or dark green color. These include kale, squash, peppers, carrots, turnip greens green onions, sweet potatoes, collards, spinach, and romaine lettuce, among others. You should eat these foods often because research demonstrates that vitamin A can protect against cancer and immune problems. In women who are prone to allergies and infections, sufficient vitamin A intake can help bolster immune protection by strengthening the cell walls and mucous membranes. This protects against developing respiratory disease, as well as allergic episodes. In addition, research has linked low vitamin A levels to breast cancer, lung cancer, cervical cancer, bladder cancer, prostate cancer, and benign breast disease.

Vitamin A can play an important role in maintaining the health of women during their menopausal transition and postmenopausal years. One study from the University of South Africa found that women with heavy menstrual bleeding (a common problem as women transition into menopause) had lower blood vitamin A levels than normal volunteers.

Other studies suggest that a high intake of beta-carotene containing foods protects against heart attacks in high-risk people. *The Nurse's Health Study*, sponsored by Harvard University Medical School found that women consuming 15 to 20 mg per day of beta-carotene had a 40 percent lower risk of strokes and a 22 percent lower risk of heart attacks when compared to women consuming less than 6 mg per day. Vitamin A deficiency has also been linked to fatigue, night blindness, skin aging, loss of smell, loss of appetite, and softening of bones and teeth.

Many vegetables are high in vitamin C. These include Brussels sprouts, broccoli, cauliflower, kale, peppers, parsley, peas, and tomatoes. Vitamin C helps to strengthen capillaries and prevent capillary fragility, thereby facilitating the flow of essential nutrients throughout the body and the excretion of waste products out of the body. This is particularly important for women transitioning into menopause who are prone to heavy menstrual bleeding.

When used in combination with foods containing bioflavonoids like soy, alfalfa, and buckwheat, foods high in vitamin C can actually help decrease menstrual flow. Vitamin C is also an important anti-stress vitamin because it is needed for healthy adrenal hormone production (the adrenal glands help us deal with stress). This is especially important for women with anxiety due to emotional causes, allergies, or stress from other origins. Vitamin C is important for immune function and wound healing. Its anti-infectious properties may help to reduce the tendency toward respiratory, bladder, and vaginal infections. Research also suggests that along with vitamin A, vitamin C may help protect women from developing cervical cancer.

Vegetables are also outstanding foods for their high mineral content. Many vegetables are high in calcium, magnesium, and potassium, which help to relieve and prevent the symptoms of menstrual cramps and PMS. Besides helping to relax tense muscles, these minerals also calm the emotions. Both calcium and magnesium act as natural tranquilizers, a benefit for women suffering from menstrual pain, discomfort, and irritability. Potassium aids in relieving the symptoms of premenstrual bloating by reducing fluid retention. These minerals are found in abundance in bone and help to provide strength to our bones. They also help to regulate the electrical activity of the heart and provide alkalinity to the body.

As you can see, calcium, magnesium and potassium are very important minerals for the overall health of our bodies. Some of the best sources for these minerals include potatoes, broccoli, kale, Swiss chard, spinach, beet greens, mustard greens, sweet potatoes, peas, and green beans. These vegetables are also high in iron, which may also help to reduce cramps. In addition, the calcium, magnesium, potassium, and iron found in vegetables also help protect against the development of anemia, osteoporosis, and excessive menstrual bleeding.

These minerals can also increase and maintain energy levels. Calcium, magnesium, and potassium help to improve stamina, endurance, and vitality. Clinical studies have shown that supplemental magnesium and potassium reduce depression and increase energy levels dramatically. Iodine and trace minerals are essential for healthy thyroid function and thus, maintaining a steady energy level; vegetables like kelp and other types of seaweed are high in these minerals.

Vegetables contain not only high levels of vitamins and minerals, but also other chemicals that help prevent heart attacks and boost immune function. Onions and garlic decrease blood clotting and lower serum cholesterol, which can de-crease the incidence of stroke and heart attack. Garlic has also been found to prevent and slow tumor growths in animals. Studies indicate that ginger root, onions, and mushrooms may have a similar effect. Certain mushrooms may even stimulate immune function. Vegetables like broccoli and cauliflower contain chemicals called indoles and isothiocyanates, which help block the activation of carcinogens, such as tobacco smoke, before they cause harm the body.

Green leafy vegetables like spinach, kale and collard greens contain essential antioxidants like lutein and zeaxanthin, which reduce your risk of macular degeneration. Lutein is also necessary for healthy ovulation and progesterone production in women thereby helping to reduce estrogen dominance in the premenopause transition. It also reduces the risk of cardiovascular disease. I usually eat a serving of green leafy vegetables every single day for their health benefits!

Vegetable Groups

Root Vegetables
Beets
Carrots
Garlic
Onions
Radishes
Rutabagas
Turnips

Cruciferous Vegetables
Broccoli
Brussels sprouts
Cabbage
Cauliflower

Gourds
Acorn squash
Butternut squash
Chayote
Crook-neck
Squash
Cucumber
Pumpkin
Zucchini squash

Nightshades
Chili pepper
Eggplant
Garden pepper
Paprika
Potatoes
Sweet potatoes
Tomatoes

Leafy Greens
Chard
Kale
Lettuce
Collard greens
Spinach
Dandelion greens

Mushrooms
Button
Shiitake

7

Nutritional Supplements For Fasting and Detoxification Programs

I recommend taking a vitamin and mineral supplement that contains a wide variety of antioxidants while doing a detoxification diet or fasting. During this time, your body will be metabolizing and eliminating large amount of toxic waste products. B vitamins are very important for your detoxification capacity. Supplemental vitamins and minerals will support both the repair of your liver and help restore your liver to optimal functioning.

Protect Your Liver Through Antioxidants

The health of the liver depends on having sufficient levels of antioxidants in the liver tissue to scavenge free radicals that interfere with liver functioning. A free radical is a type of oxygen molecule that freely moves inside cells, reacting with proteins, fats, and DNA, changing their structure and disrupting their functions.

Free radicals are generated by the metabolism of oxygen and other chemicals, including unsaturated fats, cigarette smoke, environmental chemicals, food additives, and even by aerobic exercise. It's estimated that about seventeen percent of our total oxygen consumption turns into free radicals.

The process of detoxification itself also generates a certain amount of free radicals as by-products of the chemical reactions involved, and an accelerated detoxification process, such as that which occurs during a modified fast or cleansing program, will generate even higher levels of free radicals than normal. As a result, free radicals can cause an extreme amount of damage within our bodies.

Antioxidants help to protect us from free radical damage. Antioxidants unite with free radicals and deactivate them, preventing them from doing damage. You might also want to add antioxidant rich foods and juices to your diet while doing a detoxification diet or modified fasting. These include super antioxidant fruits like pomegranate, acai berries, mangosteen, and blueberries; leafy green vegetables like kale and collard greens; as well as many other fruits and vegetables. These antioxidant rich fruits and vegetables are, of course, beneficial for us to include in our diet throughout the year!

B-Complex Vitamins

The vitamin B complex includes thiamine (B1), riboflavin (B2), niacin (B3), pantothenic acid (B5), vitamin B6, vitamin B12, folic acid, biotin, choline, and inositol. They are water-soluble and are not stored well in the body, requiring that some be consumed each day, in food or supplements. People who eat a diet of mostly processed foods high in white sugar and flour, as well as those who consume a lot of alcohol, need greater amounts of B-complex vitamins. B complex vitamins are important for healthy detoxification by the liver.

The richest source of B vitamins is brewer's yeast, but other good sources include the germ and bran of cereal grains and animal liver. Some B vitamins are also made in the intestines. Antibiotics such as sulfa drugs and tetracycline can interfere with this production, so when taking medications such as these, it is important to supplement your diet. B vitamins are critical for the production of energy within the cells and are also vital for the metabolism of fats.

The B vitamins play many roles in maintaining the health of the liver. They are vital for the deactivation of excess hormones, including estrogen, which was initially documented in studies by Morton S. Biskind in the early 1940s. Biskind found that a number of B vitamins were necessary to prevent female health issues related to estrogen dominance.

Thiamine is needed for the metabolism of alcohol to degrade it to nontoxic carbon dioxide and water. Animal studies indicate that niacin protects against carbon tetrachloride poisoning and lowers cholesterol and triglyceride levels in the blood. And folic acid and vitamin B12 have been shown to counteract fatty liver (accumulation of fat within the liver).

Vitamin B deficiencies are common factors in most liver diseases. The treatment of alcoholic liver disease, for example, requires supplementation with thiamine, vitamin B6, and folic acid. Macrocytic anemia, which is associated with liver disease, requires folic acid and vitamin B12.

Suggested Dosage: A standard dose for most B-complex nutritional supplements is between 25 and 100 mg per day. (However, some of the nutrients contained within these products, like folic acid, biotin, and B12, are included in smaller amounts, measured in micrograms.)

In summary, it is very important to support your liver with antioxidant supplements such as vitamins C, E, beta-carotene and selenium. As mentioned, the full range of B vitamins is also very important for healthy liver function. High quality nutritional supplements that contain optimal levels of these antioxidants and other essential nutrients are readily available in health food stores and many super-markets as well as through the Internet.

If you experience digestive distress from vitamin and mineral supplements during the time that you are fasting, you can cut down the dosage or eliminate them during the period of the fast, as long as the fast is not prolonged (over 2 weeks.)

Sample Nutritional Supplement Formula

I provide a sample vitamin and mineral formula that can be used as a basic foundation. It is rich in antioxidants and other nutrients like B vitamins that are essential for liver health and for efficient detoxification.

This sample formula is typical of the better quality multi-nutrient products that are available in health food stores and through the Internet. Remember that all individuals differ somewhat in their nutritional needs. If you do take vitamin or herbal supplements, I usually advise that you start with one-fourth to one-half the dose recommended in this book and work your way up slowly to the higher dosage, if needed. You may find that you do best with slightly more or less of certain ingredients.

I usually recommend that my patients take their supplements with meals or at least a snack. Very rarely, a woman will have a digestive reaction to supplements, such as nausea or indigestion. If this happens, stop all supplements; then resume using them, adding one at a time, until you find the offending nutrient. Eliminate from your program any nutrient to which you have a reaction. If you have any specific questions about the advisability of using supplemental nutrients, it is important that you ask a health-care professional who is knowledgeable about nutrition.

Sample Nutritional Supplementation for General Health and Detoxification

Vitamins and Mineral	Maximum Daily Dose
Vitamin A	5000 I.U.
Beta carotene (provitamin A)	10,000 – 25,000 I.U.
Vitamin B complex	
B1 (thiamine)	25 - 100 mg
B2 (riboflavin)	25 - 100 mg
B3 (niacinamide)	25 - 100 mg
B5 (pantothenic acid)	25 - 100 mg
B6 (pyridoxine)	50 – 100 mg
B12 (cyanocobalamin)	50 – 250 mg
Folic acid	400 – 800 mcg
Biotin	200 mcg
Choline	25 - 100 mcg
Inositol	25 - 100 mcg
PABA	25 - 100 mcg
Vitamin C (as mineral ascorbates)	1000-2000 mg
Vitamin D	1000 I.U.
Bioflavonoids	800-2000 mg
Rutin	200 mg
Vitamin E (d-alpha tocopherol acetate)	800-1600 I.U.
Calcium	1000 - 1200 mg
Magnesium	500 - 600 mg
Potassium	100 mg
Iron	18 mg
Zinc	15 mg
Iodine	150 mcg
Manganese	5 mg
Copper	2 mg
Selenium	200 mcg
Chromium	100 – 200 mcg
Boron	3 mg

Green Food Supplements

While going on a modified fast or juice fast, you may want to additional green foods to your detoxification program. Green foods are important ingredients in detoxification and cleansing programs because when, which imparts the green color to these foods, helps to neutralize and remove toxins. The greener the plant, the greater the amount of chlorophyll it contains. Foods high in chlorophyll provide energy, help heal digestive disorders, boost immunity, and prevent deficiency diseases such as anemia. Certain grasses and algae, which are described below, are especially high in chlorophyll.

As cited in an article published in *Mutation Research*, the National Institute for Occupational Safety and Health estimated that several millions workers from the manufacturing industry have been exposed to potentially hazardous chemicals, many of which cause genetic mutation and promote cancer.

This same article reports on a study that shows the effectiveness of chlorophyll in counteracting the mutagenic effect of pollutants like cigarette smoke, coal dust, and diesel-emission particles. Chlorophyll was extremely effective at inhibiting the mutations of the various aromatic amines, nitrogen compounds, and hydrocarbons found in these substances.

Chlorophyll protected against harmful compounds in fried beef and pork, red grape juice, and red wine as well. Chlorophyll has also been used successfully to treat iron deficiency anemia when used with iron supplements and peptic ulcers.

Pure extracted liquid chlorophyll is available in local health food stores. Always use chlorophyll that has been extracted from alfalfa or other plants; avoid the chemically manufactured variety. There is a benefit to consuming the plant itself as a source of chlorophyll, since grasses and algae offer their own additional properties. **Suggested Dosage**: 100 mg capsules two or three times a day. It is also available in liquid form.

Wheat Grass and Barley Grass

Cereal grasses, such as wheat grass and barley grass, are high-chlorophyll foods. Commercially, they are available fresh and as supplements, in both powder and tablet form. It is also possible to grow wheat grass at home. Both have nearly identical therapeutic properties, although barley grass may be digested a little more easily by some. People with allergies to wheat and other cereals can usually tolerate these grasses since grain in its grass stage rarely triggers an allergic reaction. These grasses contain about the same quotient of protein as meat, about 20 percent, as well as vitamin B12, chlorophyll, vitamin A, and many other nutrients.

Wheat grass is capable of incorporating more than 90 out of the estimated possible 102 minerals found in rich soil. Wheat and barley grasses have been used to treat hepatitis and high cholesterol, as well as arthritis, peptic ulcers, and hypoglycemia. They are both effective in reducing inflammation and contain the antioxidant superoxide dismutase (SOD), which slows cellular deterioration, plus various digestive enzymes that aid in detoxification.

Suggested Dosage: Combine 1-2 tbsp. of the powder or 1-2 oz. of the fresh juice in 8 oz. of water.

Microalgae

Spirulina, chlorella, and wild blue-green algae have more chlorophyll than any other foods. These algae are aquatic plants, spiral-shaped and emerald to blue-green in color, and have been used medicinally for thousands of years in South America and Africa. Today they can be purchased, in dried powder form, in health food stores.

They are also the highest sources of protein, beta-carotene, and nucleic acids of any animal or plant food, as well as containing the essential fatty acids omega-3 and gamma linolenic acid. The protein in spirulina and chlorella is so easily digested and absorbed that two or three teaspoons of these microalgae are equivalent to two to three ounces of meat. Further, unlike animal protein, the protein in algae generates a minimum of waste products when it is metabolized, thereby lessening stress on the liver.

Spirulina. Spirulina detoxifies the kidneys and liver, inhibiting the growth of fungi, bacteria, and yeasts. Because spirulina is so easily digested, it yields quick energy. It is strongly anti-inflammatory and therefore useful in the treatment of hepatitis, gastritis, and other inflammatory diseases. Spirulina strengthens body tissues and protects the vascular system by lowering blood fat. Athletes use spirulina for energy and for its cleansing action after strenuous physical exertion, which can stimulate the body to rid itself of poisons.

Suggested Dosage: A standard dosage of spirulina is 1 to 2 tbsp. stirred into 8 oz. of water per day. Green foods are very concentrated, so start with a half dose and increase gradually to make sure it's tolerated well.

Chlorella. This well-known algae is a particularly effective detoxifier as well as anti-inflammatory agent because it has high levels of chlorophyll, which stimulates these processes. Chlorella is notable for its tough outer cell walls, which bind with heavy metals, pesticides, and carcinogens such as PCBs (polychlorinated biphenyls) and then carry these toxins out of the body. This algae also promotes growth and repair of all kinds of tissue, because of chlorella growth factor. Animal research studies show that it also reduces cholesterol and atherosclerosis.

Suggested Dosage: 1 tbsp. taken in 8-12 oz. of water. Green foods are very concentrated. Be sure to begin with a partial dose and increase gradually.

Wild blue-green algae. Wild blue-green algae grows in Klamath Lake in Oregon and is processed by freeze-drying. It is sold under various trade names, frequently as a mail-order product. Wild blue-green algae is especially energizing and can improve an individual's mental concentration. However, a sign of overuse is weakness and a lack of mental focus, and certain forms are known to be highly toxic.

Many of my female patients who are in their late thirties and forties report that taking blue-green algae helps lessen the fatigue and mood swings associated with PMS and perimenopausal hormone imbalances. While I have not found it to be helpful in reducing physical symptoms such as bloating, breast tenderness, and menstrual irregularity, it does seem to promote more efficient liver function.

Since the liver has a crucial role in detoxifying and deactivating estrogen, healthy liver function helps to bring estrogen levels into balance, thereby relieving the fatigue, depression, and moodiness often found in perimenopausal women.

Suggested Dosage: 1 tbsp. daily in 8 to 12 oz. of water. It is important to buy wild blue-green algae from a reputable company that processes the algae in an FDA-approved laboratory. To avoid certain wild blue-green algae that is highly toxic, never collect it yourself or consume any that you have gathered.

Various green foods can be combined in an easy-to-digest, highly nutritious drink, which is very helpful while on a detoxification and cleansing program. As with all concentrated foods, begin with small amounts and work up to your final level.

8

Delicious Recipes for Detoxification Diet and Juice Fasting

In this chapter, I share with you 60 scrumptious and healthy recipes that promote healthy detoxification and support healing of the liver and entire body. You can use these recipes as guidelines for your own menu planning. You can use them just as they are or modify them to your own taste. I hope that you enjoy them!

Recipes for Juice Fasting

Juice Maker Recipes

Using any good quality juice maker should work well for the majority of these recipes. Juicing is a great way to enjoy and benefit from a large serving of healthy, fresh vegetables and fruits. I recommend drinking your juice on an empty stomach. The amount of juice produced from each recipe is an approximation since the size and water content of the produce can vary greatly.

Colorful Carrot Juice   Makes 2 cups

5 carrots
¼ cup fresh parsley
1 beet
2 stalks celery

Juice the carrots, beets, parsley, and celery.
Serve immediately.

Green Goddess   Makes 2 cups

*The spinach gives you a healthy serving of greens and the
lemon provides additional vitamin C.*

4 carrots
3 cups spinach
1 cucumber
4 stalks celery
½ lemon

Juice the carrots, spinach, cucumber, celery, and
lemon. Serve immediately.

Super Green   **Makes 2 cups**

This is my favorite juice drink. The ginger gives it a spicy flavor and the apple adds a little bit of sweetness. Kale is also one of the most nutrient rich vegetables and an excellent source of calcium and lutein, which supports the health of your vision.

1 bunch of kale
1 cucumber
3 stalks of celery
1 granny smith apple
½ lemon
1 tablespoon fresh ginger

Juice the kale, cucumber, celery, apple, lemon and ginger. Serve immediately.

Carrot Apple Zinger   **Makes 2 cups**

5 carrots
1 apple, red or green
1 beet
2 celery stalks
1 tablespoon fresh ginger

Juice the carrots, apple, beet, celery, and ginger. Serve immediately.

Carrot Apple Juice   Makes 2 cups

This simple drink is sweet and delicious.

5 carrots,
2 apples
½ lime, peeled

Juice the carrots, apple, and lime. Serve immediately.

Sunshine Juice   Makes 1½ cups

This drink makes a beautiful butter yellow. I enjoy this juice because it is delicate and refreshing. The fennel bulb, stalk, and leaves are all edible and fennel contains substantial amounts of vitamin C.

1 fennel bulb
2 golden beets
1 large green apple

Juice the fennel bulb, beets, and apple.
Serve immediately.

Watercress and Apple   Makes 1-1½ cups

Watercress is a tart and spicy green rich in chlorophyll. Please note that if you have a sensitive stomach be careful with watercress as it is very strong. It is recommended to start with a smaller amount of watercress and add more as your stomach becomes accustomed to it.

½ cup watercress
2 large green apples
½ cup cucumber
¼ lemon, no peel (optional)

Juice the watercress, apples, cucumber, and lemon. Serve immediately.

Super Spinach   Makes 1½-2 cups

5 cups spinach (washed very well)
1 cup red grapes
1 cup cucumber
2 cups carrot

Juice the spinach, red grapes, cucumber and carrots. Serve immediately.

Grapefruit Zinger   Makes 1½ cups

6 carrots
½-1 grapefruit, no skin
½ inch piece of ginger

Juice the carrots, grapefruit, and ginger.
Serve immediately.

Carrot Ginger   Makes 1 cup

6 carrots
½ inch piece of ginger

Juice the carrots and ginger. Serve immediately.

Note: If you prefer more spiciness add slightly more ginger

Fabulous Fennel Apple   Makes 2½ cups

1 apple
4 carrots
2 cups fennel
½ lemon, no peel, no pith
½ inch piece ginger

Juice the apple, carrots, fennel, lemon and ginger.
Serve immediately.

Carrot Fennel   Makes 2½-3 cups

8-10 carrots
1 fennel bulb with greens

Juice the carrots and fennel. Serve immediately.

Grapefruit Cleanser   Makes 2 cups

2 apples
1 grapefruit
2 celery stalks

Juice the apples, grapefruit and celery stalks. Serve immediately.

Note: Grapefruit can be a little pulpy and I recommend alternating juicing the grapefruit with the firmer apples and celery.

Liver Cleanser   Makes 1 cup

6-8 carrots
1 cup dandelion greens
1 cup kale
½ lemon

Juice the carrots, dandelion greens, kale and lemon. Serve immediately.

Note: Dandelion root is delicious and healthy but also strong in flavor, a little goes a long way.

Apple Carrot Cleanser   Makes 1½-2 cups

6-8 carrots
½ green apple
½ cup dandelion greens
1 cup kale
½ lemon

Juice the carrots, apple, dandelion greens, kale and lemon. Serve immediately.

Cleansing Apple Zinger   Makes 1½ cups

2 green apples
½ cup dandelion greens
½ inch piece of ginger
¼ cup fresh mint

Juice the apples, dandelion greens, ginger and mint. Serve immediately.

Refreshing Grape Cleanser   Makes 1 cup

1 cup red grapes
1 carrot
½ dandelion greens
¼ cup mint

Juice the grapes, carrot, dandelion greens and mint. Serve immediately.

Vegetable Juice Cocktail   Serves 4

A healthy twist on a classic. This drink uses purchased organic tomato juice with the freshly juiced vegetables adding additional nutrients. Simply juice the vegetables and add to the tomato juice.

2 cups organic low-sodium tomato or vegetable juice
2 cups spinach
4 carrots
2 stalk of celery
½ green pepper
1 cucumber
¼ cup parsley
½ lemon, peeled
¼ teaspoon paprika

Juice the spinach, cucumber, carrots, celery, lemon, green pepper, and parsley. Combine with tomato juice. Add paprika, and stir well. Garnish with celery stalks and serve right away.

Blenderized Juices

Mega Green   Makes 2½ cups

1 cup kale
1 Granny Smith apple
½ cucumber
1 cup water or apple juice

Variation: add a few sprigs of mint

Add all ingredients to a blender and liquefy on high speed. Serve immediately.

Tropical Green   Makes 2½ -3 cups

1 cup kale
1 pear
½ papaya
1 cup water

Add all ingredients to a blender and liquefy on high speed. Serve immediately.

Orange Sunset   Makes 2 cups

1 orange
½ carrot
½ papaya
1 cup water or orange juice

Add all ingredients to a blender and liquefy on high speed. Serve immediately.

Watermelon Bliss   Makes 3 cups

1 cup watermelon
1 apple
½ cup cucumber
1 cup water or apple juice

Add all ingredients to a blender and liquefy on high speed. Serve immediately.

Refreshing Melon   Makes 3 cups

1 cup watermelon
1 pear
½ cup cucumber
1 cup water or apple juice
Few mint leaves

Add all ingredients to a blender and liquefy on high speed. Serve immediately.

Recipes for Modified Fasting and Detoxification Diets

Power Smoothies

Raspberry Flax Smoothie   Serves 2

This creamy smoothie makes a great breakfast. Flaxseed oil one is my favorite foods. It is both delicious and rich in healthy omega 3 fatty acids. It also adds extra creaminess to the smoothie.

1 cup rice milk
⅔ cup raspberries – fresh or frozen
1 heaping tablespoon rice protein powder
1 tablespoon flaxseed oil
2 bananas, sliced

Combine all ingredients in a blender. Puree until smooth and serve.

Blueberry Coconut Smoothie   Serves 2

1 cup coconut water
⅔ cup blueberries – fresh or frozen
1 heaping tablespoon raw coconut flour
1 heaping tablespoon raw almonds (10-15)
1 banana, sliced

Combine all ingredients in a blender. Puree until smooth and serve.

Peachy Flax Smoothie   Serves 2

If you are using frozen peaches, chopping the peaches beforehand will reduce the puree time in the blender.

½ cup orange juice
½ cup unsweetened rice milk
1 cup peaches – fresh or frozen
1 tablespoon rice protein powder
2 teaspoons ground flaxseed
1 banana, sliced

Combine all ingredients in a blender. Puree until smooth and serve.

Strawberry Coconut Smoothie   Serves 2

This drink fits its name! It is absolutely scrumptious as well as good for you. If you don't have a high-speed blender and you are using whole raw cashews I recommend that you chop them up beforehand. Otherwise, raw cashew butter is a good substitute.

1 cup coconut milk, unsweetened
1 cup strawberries – fresh or frozen
1 tablespoon raw coconut flour
1 tablespoon raw cashews (about cashews 10-15)
1 banana, sliced

Combine all ingredients in a blender. Puree until smooth and serve.

Pomegranate Strawberry Smoothie   Serves 2

½ cup coconut water
½ cup pomegranate juice
1 cup strawberries – fresh or frozen
1 heaping tablespoon coconut flour
1 banana, sliced

Combine all ingredients in a blender. Puree until smooth and serve.

Blueberry Pomegranate Smoothie   Serves 2

¼ cup nondairy yogurt, unsweetened
¾ cup pomegranate juice
1 cup blueberries, fresh or frozen
1 tablespoon ground flaxseed
1 banana

Combine all ingredients in a blender. Puree until smooth and serve.

Delicious Green Drink   Serves 1

½ cup Concord grape juice
¼ cup water
1 tablespoon ground flaxseed
½ teaspoon chlorella powder
½ teaspoon spirulina powder

Mix all ingredients together in a glass or puree in a blender.

Gorgeous Yogurt Flax Smoothie   Serves 2

Ground flaxseed is one of my favorite breakfast additions. It blends beautifully in shakes and creates a very nice, thick consistency. Truvia is a stevia-based sweetener that has a sugar-like texture and flavor without the calories of sugar.

2 tablespoons ground flaxseed
½ cup unsweetened soy yogurt
2 cups nondairy milk
2 bananas
1 packet of Truvia
Pinch of cinnamon

Combine all ingredients in a blender. Puree until smooth and serve.

Blueberry and Greens Shake   Serves 2

This drink is a powerhouse of nutrients! The chlorella and spirulina are highly beneficial green foods. They are rich in nutrients like beta-carotene and help to detoxify the liver. They are readily available at health food stores.

1 cup nondairy milk
⅔ cup blueberries – fresh or frozen
2 tablespoons protein powder
½ teaspoon chlorella
½ teaspoon spirulina
Sprinkle of Truvia (optional)

In a blender puree the nondairy milk and blueberries. Add rest of ingredients and blend well.

Simple Flax Smoothie   Serves 1

Flaxseed is not only a tasty addition to smoothies but it is also very nutritious. Flaxseed is high in essential fatty acids, calcium, magnesium, and potassium.

1 cup vanilla nondairy milk
2 tablespoons ground flaxseed
1 banana

Combine all ingredients in a blender. Blend until smooth and serve.

Raspberry Yogurt Smoothie   Serves 2

¼ cup nondairy yogurt
1 cup raspberries – fresh or frozen
¾ cup rice milk
1 banana
2 teaspoons protein powder
Sprinkle of Truvia (if desired)

Combine all ingredients in a blender. Puree until smooth and serve.

Light Soups

Split Pea Soup   Serves 4

¾ cup split peas
5 cups low-sodium chicken broth
⅔ cup carrot, chopped
¾ cup onion, diced
Tamari soy sauce – to taste (optional)

Bring the water to a boil and add the split peas,
onion, carrots, and bouillon cubes. Reduce heat to
low and simmer for 50 minutes – 1 hour, stirring
occasionally. If water begins to cook off add up to an
extra cup of water. Add a dash of tamari soy sauce
for a saltier flavor.

Black Bean Soup   Serves 4

This recipe is easy and makes a delicious, filling soup.

1 can black beans (14 ounce), rinsed
5 cups low-sodium vegetable broth
1 cup onion, diced
⅔ cup carrot, chopped
⅔ cup red pepper, chopped
¼ teaspoon cumin
Tamari soy sauce – to taste (optional)

Bring the water to a boil and add all ingredients.
Reduce heat to low and simmer for 30 minutes,
stirring occasionally. If water begins to cook off add
up to one extra cup of water. Add a dash of tamari
soy sauce for a saltier flavor.

Vegetable Soup   Serves 4 to 6

1 onion, chopped
1 stalk celery, chopped
1 turnip, chopped
½ leek, chopped
2 carrots, chopped
¼ bunch parsley, chopped
5 mushrooms, sliced
½ tablespoon fennel
1 bay leaf
½ tablespoon thyme
1 ½ quarts vegetable broth

Place all ingredients in a pot. Cover with the vegetable broth from the previous recipe. Bring to a boil, then turn heat to low. Cook for 35-45 minutes. Pour the soup into individual serving dishes.

Summer Squash Soup   Serves 6

4 yellow summer squash
1 quart water
1 onion, chopped
½ teaspoon tamari soy sauce

Place chopped squash and onion in a pot. Add the water, bring to a boil and then turn heat to low and cover pot. Cook for 15 minutes over low flame. Add tamari soy sauce and continue cooking for another 15 minutes, until vegetables are soft. Let cool and then purée in blender. Garnish with sliced scallions or minced parsley.

Butternut Squash Soup   Serves 4

This soup has been a long-time favorite of mine. I adore the light, creamy texture. Adding maple syrup enhances the natural sweetness of the squash.

½ onion, diced
1 cup low-sodium chicken broth
2 cups butternut squash- fresh, frozen, or canned (fresh is preferred)
½ teaspoon cinnamon
1 ½ cups nondairy milk
1-2 tablespoons maple syrup
1 tablespoon safflower oil
½-¾ teaspoon salt

In a large saucepan heat the oil on medium heat. Add the onion and cook until translucent. Add the butternut squash, chicken broth, cinnamon and salt. Mix well and simmer for 5 minutes. Add nondairy milk and maple syrup. Simmer on low heat for ten minutes. Stir frequently while cooking the soup.

Optional: To make extra creamy, blend the soup when it has finished cooking. Wait for the soup to cool before blending.

Salads

Radicchio and Orange Salad   Serves 4-6

This is a sophisticated and delicious salad. I love salads with extras such as fruit.

6 cups salad greens
½ radicchio, sliced thin
¼ red onion, sliced very thin
1 medium sized orange, peeled and cut into bite size segments
Lemon juice and olive oil – to taste

In a large bowl combine salad greens, onion, oranges, and radicchio. Add the lemon juice and olive oil and toss the salad. Serve immediately.

Watercress Salad   Serves 4

8 cups mixed greens
1 ½ cups watercress, stems removed
½ cup cucumber, chopped
1 medium tomato, chopped
2 teaspoons scallion, finely chopped
Lemon juice and olive oil – to taste

Rinse the mixed greens and watercress. Remove the large stems and place in a bowl. Add the cucumber, tomatoes, and scallions. Add the lemon juice and olive oil and toss the salad. Serve immediately.

Scrumptious Veggie Salad   Serves 4-6

This is one of my favorite salads! It pairs wonderfully with soups and sandwiches

1 head red lettuce, chopped into bite size pieces
1 large tomato, chopped
2 green onions, sliced
6 mushrooms, sliced
¾ cup kidney beans – canned works well
Lemon juice and olive oil – to taste

Combine all ingredients in a large salad bowl. Add the lemon juice and olive oil and toss the salad. Serve immediately.

Wild Rice and White Bean Salad   Serves 4

6 ounces great northern or navy beans
2 cups cooked wild rice
3 scallions, chopped
¼ to ½ cup minced parsley
½ green pepper, minced
Lemon juice and olive oil – to taste

Combine all the ingredients in a bowl. Mix with lemon juice and olive oil to taste.

Note: Brown rice may be substituted for wild rice.

Brown Rice and Black Bean Salad   Serves 4

2 cups cooked brown rice
1 cup black beans, cooked
1 green onion, diced
¼ cup raisins
¼ cup peas, cooked
¼ cup green pepper
¼ cup celery
Lemon or lime juice and olive oil – to taste

Combine all ingredients in a bowl. The salad may be dressed with lemon or lime juice and olive oil.

Lentil Salad   Serves 4

1 cup lentils
3 cups water
½ teaspoon sea salt
¼ cup celery, finely chopped
¼ cup red onion, finely chopped
¼ cup black olives, finely chopped
2 -3 tablespoons lemon juice
1-2 tablespoons olive oil
1 teaspoon dried basil

Wash lentils and combine with water in a pot. Cook for 30 minutes or until lentils are soft, adding more water if necessary. Combine all ingredients in a bowl. Toss with lemon juice, olive oil, and basil.

Grains

Brown Rice   Serves 4

1 cup brown rice
2 cups cold water

Wash rice with cold water. Combine all ingredients in a cooking pot. Bring ingredients to a rapid boil. Turn heat to low, cover, and cook without stirring about 25 to 35 minutes, until rice is soft.

Quinoa   Makes 2 cups

Most recipes call for a 2:1 ratio, but I prefer 1:1 ½ I find that this makes a fluffier, lighter quinoa, which I prefer.

1 cup quinoa
1 ½ cups water

Rinse quinoa and drain through a fine sieve. Boil the water and add quinoa. Turn to very low heat and cook for 20-25 minutes.

Kasha

1 cup kasha (buckwheat groats)
3 cups water

Bring ingredients to a boil, lower heat, and simmer for 15-20 minutes or until soft. The grains should be fluffy like rice.

Note: Kasha is especially good for women with PMS. For breakfast, blend in blender with water until it has a creamy texture. Toppings include: sunflower milk, almond milk, or sesame milk; and cinnamon, apple butter, ginger, raisins, or berries.

Simple Vegetable Dishes

Simple Cabbage   Serves 1

This cabbage makes a simple and nutritious side dish.

½ Savoy cabbage, cored
Pinch of salt and pepper

Wash and core the cabbage. Cut cabbage into four wedges and steam for 4-5 minutes, or until tender. Remove from pan and add a pinch of salt and pepper.

Kale with Lemon   Serves 2

Kale is one of my favorite vegetables and it also has terrific health benefits since it is a good source of calcium and other essential nutrients like lutein, which supports the health of your eyes.

1 bunch of kale
1 lemon, cut into quarters
Tamari soy sauce

Rinse kale well and remove stems. Steam for 5-6 minutes or until leaves wilt and are tender. Dress lightly with tamari soy sauce and lemon juice.

Celery Julienne   **Serves 4**

6 stalks celery
2 tablespoons sweet red pepper, chopped

Cut the celery into small strips (like french-fried potatoes). Steam for 15 to 20 minutes, or until tender. Drain and toss with red pepper.

Steamed Baby Bok Choy   **Serves 2-4**

This dish is delicious served over brown rice!

4-6 baby bok choy
Tamari soy sauce

Steam for 4 to 5 minutes or until stalks are tender. Serve with a sprinkle of tamari soy sauce.

Steamed Swiss Chard   **Serves 2-4**

1 bunch Swiss chard

Chop the Swiss chard into 2" pieces and steam for 4-5 minutes. Using the stalks is optional.

Cauliflower with Parsley   Serves 4

1 head medium cauliflower
3 to 4 tablespoons fresh parsley, finely chopped

Break the cauliflower into small flowerets. Steam for
10 minutes or until tender. Toss with fresh parsley.

Broccoli with Lemon   Serves 4

1 pound broccoli
Juice of ½ lemon

Cut the broccoli into small flowerets; steam for 5-7
minutes or until tender. Squeeze lemon juice over
broccoli.

Roasted Turnips   Serves 4

4-6 turnips, peeled (optional)
1-2 teaspoons olive oil

Preheat oven to 350 degrees. Cut turnips in quarters
and place in baking dish lined with aluminum foil (or
a lightly oiled baking dish). Drizzle olive oil over the
turnips and roast for 30-40 minutes, until fork tender.

Savory Bean Sprouts   Serves 4

1 cup chicken stock
1 ½ cups bean sprouts
1 cup mushrooms, sliced

Heat chicken stock over a low flame for 5 minutes.
Add bean sprouts and mushrooms. Simmer for 10
minutes.

Baked Sweet Potato   Serves 1-2

1 sweet potato or yam

Cut Preheat oven to 400 degrees. Poke a few holes in
your sweet potato with a fork. Wrap in aluminum
foil (optional) and bake for one hour.

Summer Squash and Peas   Serves 4

2 to 3 small summer squash, sliced or chopped
1 cup peas

Steam peas and squash together for 5-7 minutes or
until tender. Drain and serve.

Vegetable Puree

3 to 4 carrots, chopped
¼ head cabbage, chopped
1 cup peas

Steam carrots for 15 minutes, add rest of vegetables and steam another 3-5 minutes, until soft. Place in blender and purée. Slowly add water until smooth and creamy.

About Susan M. Lark, M.D.

Dr. Susan Lark is one of the foremost authorities in the fields of women's health care and alternative medicine. Dr. Lark has successfully treated many thousands of women emphasizing holistic health and complementary medicine in her clinical practice. Her mission is to provide women with unique, safe and effective alternative therapies to greatly enhance their health and well-being.

A graduate of Northwestern University Feinberg School of Medicine, she has served on the clinical faculty of Stanford University Medical School, and taught in their Division of Family and Community Medicine.

Dr. Lark is a distinguished clinician, author, lecturer and innovative product developer. She has been an innovator in the use of self-care treatments such as diet, nutrition, exercise and stress management techniques in the field of women's health. She is the author of many best-selling books on women's health. Her signature line of nutritional supplements and skin care products are available through healthydirections.com.

One of the most widely referenced physicians on the Internet, Dr. Lark has appeared on numerous radio and television shows, and has been featured in many magazines and newspapers.

She has also served as a consultant to major corporations, including the Kellogg Company and Weider Nutrition International, and was spokesperson for The Gillette Company Women's Cancer Connection.

Dr. Lark can be contacted at (650) 561-9978 to make an appointment for a consultation.

Dr. Susan's Solutions
Health Library For Women

The following books are available from iTunes, Amazon.com, Amazon Kindle, Womens Wellness Publishing and other major booksellers. Dr. Susan is frequently adding new books to her health library.

Women's Health Issues

Dr. Susan's Solutions: Healthy Heart and Blood Pressure

Dr. Susan's Solutions: Healthy Menopause

Dr. Susan's Solutions: The Anemia Cure

Dr. Susan's Solutions: The Bladder Infection Cure

Dr. Susan's Solutions: The Candida-Yeast Infection Cure

Dr. Susan's Solutions: The Cold and Flu Cure

Dr. Susan's Solutions: The Endometriosis Cure

Dr. Susan's Solutions: The Fibroid Tumor Cure

Dr. Susan's Solutions: The Irregular Menstruation Cure

Dr. Susan's Solutions: The Menstrual Cramp Cure

Dr. Susan's Solutions: The PMS Cure

Emotional and Spiritual Balance

Breathing Meditations for Healing, Peace and Joy

Dr. Susan's Solutions: The Anxiety and Stress Cure

Dr. Susan's Solutions: The Chronic Fatigue Cure

Women's Hormones

DHEA: The Fountain of Youth Hormone

Healthy, Natural Estrogens for Menopause

Pregnenolone: Your #1 Sex Hormone

Progesterone: The Superstar of Hormone Balance

Testosterone: The Hormone for Strong Bones, Sex Drive and Healthy Menopause

Diet and Nutrition

Dr. Susan Lark's Healing Herbs for Women

Dr. Susan Lark's Complete Guide to Detoxification

Enzymes: The Missing Link to Health

Healthy Diet and Nutrition for Women: The Complete Guide

Renew Yourself Through Juice Fasting and Detoxification Diets

Energy Therapies and Anti-Aging

Acupressure for Women: Relieve Symptoms of Dozens of Health Issues Through Pressure Points

Exercise and Flexibility

Stretching and Flexibility for Women

Stretching Programs for Women's Health Issues

About Womens Wellness Publishing

"Bringing Radiant Health and Wellness to Women"

Womens Wellness Publishing was founded to make a positive difference in the lives of women and their families. We are the premier publisher of print and eBooks focused on women's health and wellness. We are committed to publishing the finest quality and most comprehensive line of books that covers every area that a woman needs to create vibrant health and a joyful, fulfilling life.

Our books are written and created by the top health and wellness experts who share with you, our readers, their wisdom and extensive experience successfully treating many thousands of patients.

We encourage you to browse through our online bookstore, womenswellnesspublishing.com, as we are frequently adding new titles. Visit our Lifestyle Center and Customer Bonus Center for more exciting and helpful health and wellness information and resources.

Follow us on Facebook for the latest health tips, recipes, and all natural solutions to many women's health issues (facebook.com/wwpublishing).

We would enjoy hearing from you! Please share your success stories, comments and requests for new topics with us at yourstory@wwpublishing.com.

About Our Associate Program

We invite you to become part of the Womens Wellness Publishing Community through our Associate Program. You will have the opportunity to earn generous commissions on sales that you create through your blog, social network, support groups, community groups, school & alumni groups, friends, family or other networks.

To join the Associate Program, go to our website, womenswellnesspublishing.com, and click "Become an Associate"

We support your sales and marketing efforts by offering you and your customers:

- Free support materials with updates on all of our new book releases, promotions, and bonuses for you and your customers
- Free audio downloads, booklets, and guides
- Special discounts and sales promotions

24079798R00055

Made in the USA
Lexington, KY
04 July 2013